Closed Legs, Open Heart

By

Victoria Green

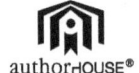

authorHOUSE®

AuthorHouse™
1663 Liberty Drive
Bloomington, IN 47403
www.authorhouse.com
Phone: 1-800-839-8640

Published by AuthorHouse 10/28/2014

ISBN: 978-1-4208-1765-2 (sc)
ISBN: 978-1-4634-5964-2 (e)

To my Father, Jehovah, and my mother, Sharlene, I am
Everything I am because you loved me.

Wholly

Untouched unused
unbroken unbruised
Resting in Whites
not
bleeding in Blues.

Unobtained untolled
unscripted unscrolled
Not Penetrated
then Frustrated
but
Virgin and Whole.

Uncounted unnamed
untaunted unashamed
Lying Vibrant and Pure
not
Exhausted and Lame.

Untaken unharmed
unhasted unswarmed
Not abused and abandoned cold
but
nurtured and secured warm.

Unopened unwronged
unissued unsung
Unmistakably Beautiful
Unbelievably Strong.

by Victoria D. Green

I. The Reason

After spending part of the summer preceding my senior year in college as a teacher and mentor for pre-teen and teenage girls, I felt confirmed and more commissioned than ever to write a book such as this. While having dialogue, lecture, and just plain eavesdropping on the casual conversation of the girls, I learned that a very large percentage of them had already engaged in sexual intercourse. When I came across this knowledge, I was more saddened than surprised, though I thoroughly experienced both emotions.

Being one who frequently finds myself in deep thought, I immediately began to ponder and meditate on what had caught my heart off guard and stung quite deeply. I was and do remain genuinely hurt for my sisters and what they have lost. I hurt for the young princesses forced from their God-given pedestals and cheated, stripped, robbed of a most precious jewel, never to be recaptured. I hurt for their lost royalty and even more at the fact that most of them are ignorant of their losses. I cry and pray for them in their brokenness; in the brokenness of their dreams, in the brokenness of their innocence, in the brokenness of their purity, in the brokenness of their **virginity.** It wasn't long before I discovered in my study that God had given me His heart, in that the very sentiments that I just shared with you were recorded as His thoughts in His Word, saying:

"When I would comfort myself against sorrow, my heart is faint in me.
Behold the cry of the daughter of my people.... For the hurt of the daughter of my people am I hurt..."
Jeremiah 8:18, 21 (KJV)

In a world where unwed, underage, and unprepared mothers are copiously existent in American society, and overpopulate and destroy the African American community, I believe such a book is imperative. When we are daily confronted with terrifying statistics about AIDS, abortions, dropout rates, suicide, and multitudes of other mishaps related to unlawful sex, I can firmly say that our world is literally dying for this book.

Firstly I would like to clarify that God is a loving, forgiving, and redeeming Father who specializes in helping us rectify, abandon, and draw strength from our mistakes. I said that to say this: The intent of this book is not to condemn sinful pasts, but to build stronger futures. We all make mistakes, but some mistakes don't have to be made and are better unmade, for that matter.

I am truly convicted to believe that as I take a deeper look at female virginity in order to highlight and salute its importance, beauty, power, and worth, that I could change minds, or at least one mind. By exposing a very intimate and passionate voice of me, I hope to make a difference. I have written this book with high hopes that some young lady will be saved from making one of the most tragic mistakes of her life and forfeiting a very special part of her being. I also wrote so that the world could know me in my virginity. So people could know that I am happy and content within myself and not agonized in choice to be abstinent. As I write unto you, do know that I am writing wholly, meaning that I still possess that unique and special gift that God has given me from birth and ordained for a proper unveiling in due time.

II. The Personal and Past

Because I have always been deemed different by my peers and superiors, or just plain different from most people in many senses, I have come to strive to be different in all that I do. This brings me to the dearest and most passionate reasons why I have vowed to maintain my virginity until marriage. Things that have happened in my past which have shaped the woman I am today have forced me to create a personal standard by which I MUST live in order to insure that I love, honor, and respect myself in the manner that I deserve.

Seeing that I am the second person in my family to attend college and the first female to matriculate and graduate from an institution of higher learning—a black Ivy League one, I might add—simply suggests that I am different. The fact that all but one of the elder females in my immediate family were unwed teenage mothers adamantly inspires and motivates me to be different. The sad truth is that the woman who brought me into this world was an unwed drug addict with four children from several different men before the age of twenty-one. I have never had a healthy relationship with her, or known her as "mother", and this strongly burdens me to be different.

Apart from the fact that I would like to think that I am a young woman of notable self-discipline, integrity, and character, there exist very personal and unique circumstances like those above that commit me to virginhood. Though I have accomplished many great things in my short life, which have gained me a host of people who look to me for encouragement, hope, inspiration, and instruction, I have also lived, loved, and learned as a partial person. This is the case because, sadly and as heartbreaking as it is, I never knew half of the partnership that is responsible for my being.

Yes, I Victoria Green, the intellect, poet, writer, minister, motivational speaker, and mentor, am also a bastard child. Even after I have found salvation and accepted my adoption into the royal family in which God is my all-protecting, providing, and prospering Father, there still lies a part of me, dormant at times, that longs to know whose blood flows through my veins. By no means am I unstable or depressed, but I do know and respect that our ability to create life is a miracle and a gift, given only by God, despite the means in which it occurs. I also know that every person should know where he or she comes from, and the lack of that knowledge causes a void in one's life, whether he or she chooses to admit it or not. I know that all things work together for my good, and God only allowed me these experiences and the deposits they left in my life in order to bring me into a time such as this, in which I would come forth to save others.

I am choosing to make the sacrifice of revealing some of the deepest and most secret parts of me in hopes that someone will be inspired, changed, or inspired to change. Though I have been noted for unusual strength, I must say that there are parts of me that hurt dearly at times. Times such as when I look at my birth certificate and there is a blank space where the father's name and information are required. Or times when I notice certain mannerisms and traits that I possess and I know that they were not attributed to me by my mother, and I wonder if they are of my father. Or when my pastor or another minister speaks about us carrying our father's seed and needing our father's blessing as cited by the Bible.

I have had and still have several exceptional male figures in my life who positively impact me, so I do not hate men or think that they are all no good. However, my experience as a bastard child has not made me weaker, but exceptionally strong. I am strong, secure, and stable within myself in regards to this information about my father, or lack thereof, and therefore I have no problem expressing it publicly. I do not consider it baggage, which most people entering relationships wish to avoid. This is the case because these circumstances do not burden me, but they have inspired me. I am successful, fulfilled, and happy, despite the fact that I know what it feels to cry yourself to sleep at night because you don't know who part of you is or where it came from, or wondering who will give you away on your wedding day.

Though I don't stress about those things anymore, now that I am a woman, I realize that I cried and wondered because I was weak as a child. I also know that there are many children out there with whom I identify, especially girls, and some of them do not make it past those weak points in their childhoods to reach the success that I have been blessed to achieve as a woman. I pray for those young girls and the women who have refused to grow because of the young, weak girls who still live inside of them. I offer myself to you through these words now. I offer my viewpoint, my experiences, my strength, and my God, and my hope to make some changes starting now. Since so many of us know what that weak, broken child feels like, why don't we commit ourselves to creating different circumstances than those that have surrounded us, to protect our future children?

Because of the many nights I have cried and wondered, I have promised myself and my unborn children that I will not lie down with any man who has not dedicated, devoted, and committed his whole self to me and the fruits of our partnership. I never want to cause a child to feel the pain that I have felt in my lifetime. Though this pain has not been crippling or an inhibitor of my growth, it was very much agonizing and avoidable. I am so passionate and convicted about breaking the cycle of creating illegitimate and parentless children in my family that I refuse to let a combination of immaturity, lack of self-restraint, and childish lust cause me to satisfy my own personal pleasure and callously birth a being into an unfit environment which could detrimentally alter his or her life forever.

III. The Spiritual

I'd like to be able to consider myself a devout Christian and seek to be a reflection of God's Excellency in all that I do. From this comes a great commandment of me to remain pure and untainted as His child. I strive to conquer great feats that will require supernatural power, which I can only draw from God and only when I exist as a pure being which He can fill. In this portion of the book, I will attempt to share my enlightenment concerning the spiritual reasoning for abstaining from premarital sex, known Biblically as fornication. I do believe that God has given me some very profound and piercing explanation on this matter, and I am motivated to inform others in hopes that someone will be impacted and changed by such eminent and finite knowledge, just as I was.

Because God has intently placed blood at the very existence and essence of human life, it is inevitable that any situation concerning the blood of one and/or another's body will affect life situations in some sense. With that in mind, and also knowing that God is not erroneous or coincidental in His actions, I have come to see the complexity of God endowing a woman with a most precious treasure which helps to define her and no earthly being could ever give her. A woman's hymen lies at the very center of her womanhood.

There is no doubt in my mind that fornication is an immoral and unhealthy act for both male and female, but my personal study and conviction just leads me to believe that the first time has to be more impacting for females. As women, the first experience of traditional sexual intercourse physically removes a part of us. Attached to the physical are also spiritual, mental, and emotional withdrawals occurring from that initial sexual experience, and each one thereafter. I wholeheartedly wish that all women could realize that in that small sack of blood buried within our physiques God has blessed us with *purity, pride*, and *power.*

In the *purity* aspect of the matter, the Father has ordained and prepared for us to be the chaste, honorable vessels that He created for his beloved sons, to remain sealed and consecrated until marriage. In the Old Testament, animal blood was offered as a sacrifice in search of atonement for sins, and only the purest blood was acceptable to God. God also provided for the ultimate sacrifice by allowing the shedding of Jesus' blood to atone for all sins. In the same sense, I can see God's charge to us to offer a sacrifice to Him, ourselves, our future husbands, and unborn children to remain pure, with our gifts untouched and unopened until His blessing allows the unveiling.

God has given us a right to *pride* in our femininity, in that He has given us a visible and tangible entrance into womanhood from a sexual viewpoint, which He has not equally endowed the male species with. Once that hymen has been torn, we have been broken by some man, whether he be Mr. Right or Mr. Right Now.

One can even see God's different interest and approach in creating the sexual beings of male and female by simply observing the two anatomies. I am moved to think of God's care and intent for us to be sexually secure in that a woman's sexual/reproductive organs are engulfed in other body parts where they are protected, hidden, and secured. On the other hand, a male's are as open, free, and unenclosed as his navel, nose, or kneecaps.

Your virginity is a jewel, and as a very special part of you, it should only be given to someone equally as special, because it should not be taken and it should not be given to just anyone who wants it or thinks they should have it. It should not be lost behind the bleachers in your high school. It should not be given away to your first boyfriend in a parked car. It should be given to someone who has pledged and proved his love (through marriage), and therefore deserves to have it. Young girls, ladies, women, queens, princesses, divas, dolls, if you don't take anything else from this book, please remember this: Sexual intercourse is very very very very deep and intimate on so many levels. When you choose to join yourself with another person and a man enters your body, he also enters your spirit. Just by looking at the blood involved in childbirth or the blood that Jesus shed on the cross, we know that the shedding of blood is a very serious issue that entails a lot in one's life. With this in mind, we should not let just any man draw blood from or enter our bodies in knowing the severity and seriousness of this circumstance.

Most importantly, God has given women **power** in our existence as virgins. Not only do we have to power to make men prove themselves worthy of having our most precious parts, but we also have the awesome power, similar to that of Jesus, to make a blood covenant. Most people know by means of the dictionary or Bible that a covenant is a partnership or agreement. My first lady even went a step further as to call it an agreement to live better, and I among others could accept that definition in seeing that all the covenants we are familiar with (Abraham, Noe, Moses, and Jesus) provided for the people to live more fulfilling lives than they had prior to the covenant.

With that said and other common knowledge, we have come to know that a blood covenant, coined by Jesus' death, is an agreement or partnership to live better and sealed by blood. We also know that covenants should not be broken, and if they are, it results in death. With those grounds laid, I can rest assured in saying that God has given us the ability or power to create a blood covenant with someone, and because God does not orchestrate covenants so that they can be broken, it should be made with your life partner (husband) and undefiled by either party.

Once you connect with a man sexually, you should have already been connected with him spiritually, emotionally, and mentally, because at this point, he is getting to know a very precious and secret part of you, which is the crown and reward for knowing you in every other manner, hence he Biblically "knows" you as Adam "knew" Eve. This scenario gives rise to the term "know" as it equates to sexual intercourse in some instances in the Bible. When your husband breaks your virginity, the two of you are merely sealing the covenant or agreement that you make each other whole, and it is an agreement that your lives are better together than they are apart. Unwed sex and loss of virginity unknowingly create many broken covenants, broken hearts, broken spirits, broken beings, and broken lives. Women, please be advised of your covenant-making power. Make sure that whoever enters into that covenant with you is worthy and committed to the covenant and not just casually stripping you of an element of your inner beauty and life.

IV. The Gift

I have previously referred to virginity and sexual intercourse as a God-given gift in other sections of the book, and I am still referring to it in the same context, but this section sheds a different light on the giver and receiver of that prized gift. When thinking of the idea expressed in this section, I often think of someone purchasing new clothes or shoes, especially white tennis shoes. Most people love a fresh pair of new white sneakers in their cleanliness and vibrancy, and though there is nothing wrong with purchasing secondhand/used items, almost everyone would prefer new things. I also believe that this is the case when men seek wives, soul mates, and girlfriends.

It is true that you can't pick whom you fall in love with, but when men have a choice or find themselves looking for that special someone, they try by all means to avoid damaged and/or used goods. What I mean by that is just as a man would prefer a brand new pair of white Air Force Ones fresh from the box, he would also be delighted with an unbroken female, fresh from God's hands. Young ladies, please beware of the fact that men have no problem using certain women for "basketball or work shoes," meaning that you are only good enough to be used by him in sex and sexual favors, but when it comes to stepping out of the house, then you're back in the box and he slides on his pearly white Reebok classics or shiny loafers and shows them off to the world. Many men will use you sexually, abuse you mentally, and neglect you socially. In laymen's terms, you can satisfy his physical desire, but you'll never be on his arm in public introduced as his lady or the love of his life.

Knowing that God has created us to someday complete some man by becoming his wife, we should be disciplined enough to not risk our destinies in premature sexual intercourse. In order to make another person whole, you must first be the whole half that you are required to be. When entering a marriage, you should do so wholly, and the mental, emotional, and spiritual scars of past sexual relationships can complicate, and in some cases terminate, the bond created in marriage. You were made for one person and one person alone, so how can he have you totally when so many people have pieces of you also? Each act of sexual intercourse takes something and adds something from your spirit to your partner's, and after so long it can be impossible to know yourself enough to pledge yourself to another.

When I think about a woman giving her virginity or sexual being to anyone other than her husband, I often analogize the scenario to the manner in which my nephew behaves on Christmas and/or his birthday. Because he is spoiled and very arrogant, he has little regard for the time, money, and effort that people must put into the purchase, preparation, and presentation of the gifts he receives. No matter how elegantly wrapped each of the presents is or what people had to go through to get them, all my nephew seems to be concerned about are the contents of the packages and whether or not they meet his approval. I've seen him callously rip through packages and discard the contents nonchalantly without even so much as a thank you, and jibe a smart remark such as "That's all" or "Next" as he awaits the next gift.

It is such a shame that so many lost boys, thinking themselves men, are ripping into our sisters' and daughters' lives with the same disregard. I hate that so many of these young women give away something that they can never get back, to people who couldn't care less about their feelings, lives, dreams, or anything else that concerns them, for as far as that goes. When you give something to someone, you cannot expect them to cherish, love, honor, and respect it if in fact they don't know the true value of it. And how can a woman effectively convey the value of herself to a man or any other person if *she* doesn't truly understand it herself ? Know the divinity of your gifts and give them only to the person who is worthy of them, because they are so very precious that another human could never create, recreate, duplicate, or restore them.

> **"Give not that which is Holy unto the
> dogs, neither cast your pearls
> Before swine, lest they trample them
> under their feet and turn again
> And rend to you" Matthew 7:6 (KJV)**

When a gift is bought or made for a particular person, then no one else should use or receive the gift except that elect person. From childhood, we know that gifts that are made versus those that are purchased are more sentimental, because they require more time, care, effort, and thought. For this reason, you should know that your virginity is a very precious and sacred gift because not only was it made, but also God Himself made it. It was made with power, precision, and passion. It was made like no other. It was made for one person. In this gift, you were given the ability by God to give your husband something that no other person could ever give him; something that you've never given another person. That is such a beautiful thing, one of the most beautiful on earth, I believe. I do believe that there is nothing greater or more special than a husband taking a virgin to bed on the wedding night. Her beauty is accented by her self-discipline and sacrifice.

It is also my belief that a woman should never lose her virginity. I say this because if your husband makes a blood covenant with you in sexual intercourse, by you losing your virginity then he is the one who has taken it.

> *"Therefore shall a man leave his father and mother, and cleave to his wife: and they shall be one flesh."*
> **Genesis 2:24 (KJV)**

Because of the fact that marriage is the concept of two becoming one, meaning also the flesh, you being one with your husband have not lost anything that you have given to him. To make the union complete, as God has commanded, you are physically joined with him following a spiritual and emotional bonding that precedes and should be a prerequisite of sexual intercourse.

V. The Truth

Condoms break and contraceptives fail, besides the fact no condom or other method of birth control can nullify the fact or validate the act of a sexual partner entering your innermost sanctum, which is exactly what happens when you engage in sex. This is the truth; it happens. It happens whether you take the pill or he wears three condoms. It happens whether he is your husband or just a guy from around the way. It happens, whether it is in the blissful warmth, security, and comfort of your honeymoon bed or in the cramped fear of a car's back seat.

If you haven't accepted or been moved by anything thus far, do know that the simple truth is you are worth the wait. The most vital elements of your existence are housed inside of your body in a special, hidden place. Among these elements is the jewel of life hoarded in the mystery of womanhood. Not everyone should be allowed to take the journey that grants access to that jewel. You are worth the wait of finding someone who will value it and every other part of you for the priceless possessions that they are. You are not a sex toy, slut, whore, tramp, or any other demeaning female misnomer. You are wife material. You are a princess of the Most High God, and in this truth, carry yourself in a royal manner, which no common man can touch or taint. The truth is, God did not take so much time and care to perfect you as a beautiful, sweet, dainty creature so that you could be misused, abused, and discarded. Know that He has crafted you as a jewel and a most peculiar one in knowing that some dynamic man should win your approval, because no ordinary man can inherit the kingdom.

A guy once asked me why we couldn't "take it to the next level"—meaning sex—and I sincerely responded with the words that I live by, "I like you, but I Love Me." I love myself and I have come to know love through sacrifice, patience, respect, and honor. I will not be added to any boy's list of conquests. I am absolutely elated at the fact that I will someday be the mother of my husband's children, but I refuse to be anybody's "baby mama."

Speaking of truth, let's be real! I am human. To be even more specific, I am a twenty-one-year-old female. I experience feelings, emotions, thoughts, and desires through temptation. At this age, my hormones are full throttle, just like any other normal young lady, but I can still stand to say that it is still very much possible to be abstinent. By no means will I say that it is easy, but with God-given restraint, it is possible to thrive in chastity and consecration. If it were not possible, our God being just, would not have called us into such beings. Though I am tempted at times to have sex, the justifications that I have rendered in this book for my abstinence are much more important than satisfying a momentary lust of my loins.

In lieu of the aforementioned contents of this book, the many circumstances in my life, thus far, have created a passion so deep in me that caused me to endeavor such a project as this book and to live the life described in it. The conditions surrounding my conception, prenatal development, and birth set the odds against me before I even entered this world. On the other hand, God was for me, and that's all I ever really needed or will ever need for that matter. Because of the things I was exposed to in the womb, I could have been born with AIDS, mentally retarded, blind, deaf, handicapped, addicted to heroin, crack, marijuana, and/or alcohol. Science says that I should have been, but God spared me. I am grateful to Him every day for that, and I'm also aware of the fact that He doesn't make miracles out of people for them to live less than extraordinary lives.

The average therapist or psychologist would probably say that I should have been an unwed teenage mother, drug addict, high school dropout, criminal, or lost in promiscuity by now. Some would even say I would have just cause to be one of the above, considering my family background and personal experience. I know what I could have or "should" have been, and because I am not, I've promised God to be different… to dedicate my life to showing people you can be different. I'm far from typical; not the average woman you'd meet these days. I'm not telling you it's easy to be different, because it is not at all, it takes a very strong person. I know and hope that you will someday know also, that this is the only reason I was created. My sole purpose on this earth is to be an instrument in showing people that by Him, things can be done that we never thought possible.

> *"But ye are a chosen generation, a royal priesthood, an holy nation, a peculiar people that you might shew forth the praises of him who hath called you out of darkness into his marvelous light."*
> **I Peter 2:9, KJV**

The above things (I have just discussed) are those that allow me to keep myself from getting into "sticky" situations. I ask God for the insight to help me make wise choices to avoid overwhelming run-ins with temptation. Because I know temptation is prevalent in all of our lives, every day that we live, I have constructed a personalized prayer, which is this:

"God give me the strength to earn my anointing, the discipline to keep it, the wisdom to use it, and the humility to maximize it."

I ask Him for the strength to earn my anointing because the Bible-backed teachings of my spiritual parents, tells me that in order to cause godly change in any area of people's lives, you must be anointed, which is to have received anointing in that area. Whether your area of ministry is drug addiction, finance, fornication and adultery, marriage, or any other area, you must receive anointing, which can only come from firsthand experience. God only gives a person anointing in specific areas when the person has proven faithful in trusting God to keep them as they suffer in that area. God answers prayers, especially when they are sincere desires to do what is right, so my prayer is, "God give me the strength to keep 'closed legs' so that my anointing will be in place to inspire women to change."

It is just as hard to keep some things as it is to get them, and anointing is surely one of those things. I know that so many spiritual leaders and beings have lost their anointing in the blink of an eye by making bad choices. I ask God for discipline to stay away from people, situations, and influences (music, movies, etc.) that might cause me to do something that will destroy my anointing, which I have spent years to earn.

I ask Him for the wisdom and humility to be teachable enough to follow His instructions concerning my ministry in this area and not think that I am better than anyone. It is easy to put myself on a pedestal compared to many women when it comes to not giving my body away, but I know complacency and pride can destroy my anointing as quickly as fornication can. I could get the big head while ministering to women and prematurely end the ministry that God has given me, which would forfeit many lives.

I pray my prayer whenever I think of it because the Bible instructs me to pray in season and out of season, which I think is a very good and relevant instruction. I say this because, as I mentioned earlier, it can be very hard at times to maintain as an abstinent, anointed woman of God. With temptation, some days are better than others, a whole lot better. Knowing this, it is important that you stay, as the old folks say, "prayed up." This means say prayers in advance or keep them stored up because you'll find that things can heat up so quickly sometimes in situations that you won't have the time or the mind to pray, if you know what I mean! Even though God has allowed me to become wiser through my journey in womanhood and adulthood, I have found myself in a few of these "heated situations."

The truth is, I have been naïve enough to think that I could handle myself in certain situations or around certain people, only to find that I couldn't and was on the verge of losing my anointing along with the significant impact that could be made on so many female lives. I know that it was only God, in response to those "stored up" prayers I mentioned, who touched me just in time, before someone else touched me!

Most of the time, I am mindful enough of my mission to keep myself in line, but there are also times where I feel someone has got to be playing games with me. I mean, some days it seems that all I come across are attractive, available men all day long and my imagination wants to run wild. Or some days I'm extra sensitive and all it takes is for someone to touch my hand, give me a friendly hug, or come close enough for me to smell his cologne, and I'm in trouble!

With this said, I urge you to do all you can to keep yourself free of "sticky situations," but when you can't help it and you somehow find yourself in one, pray a sincere prayer. It doesn't have to be my prayer, it can be "I can do all things through Christ..." or whatever works for you, as long as it's not something as inane and self-gratifying as "God, don't let me get pregnant doing this" or "Please don't let me catch anything." And oh yeah, when you're about to go too far and you begin praying, don't think that God is going to rescue you or give you strength to walk away when you're not exerting any effort or truly for real. What I mean by this is don't ask God to help you if you are continuing to willingly come out of your panties, or letting him nibble on your neck as you pray to God. God has given you free will and if you have sense enough to pray, you have sense enough to meet Him halfway.

Ladies, the truth is, if he loves you, he can wait. If he waits, the love will become stronger. With closed legs, you can open your heart and learn the meaning of true love. You can learn God's unmatched love for you and thereby learn to love yourself better than any man could ever love you so that when the time is right you will be able to love wholly. True love is worth working and waiting for.

About The Author

Victoria Green started writing in her early youth, but developed a passion for it in high school. Her poetry and short hand prose were published in several local publications in her hometown as well as elicited invitations to public and motivational speaking engagements during the initial stages of her writing career. While in college, she was deemed a Famous Poet's Poet of the Year and completed her first volume of poetry, The Divine Light, and another non-fiction title, both soon to be published. Ms. Green recently received her B.A. degree in Economics from historic Spelman College. She is currently working as a financial services representative and forever operating in her livelihood as a master of words in the capacities of writer, teacher, motivational speaker, and minister.